AF812431

American College of Surgeons
Protocol for Cancer Surgery Documentation: Lung Cancer

Name: ACS.CSSP.protocol.lung.2023.v1

What This Protocol Includes and Covers

- A synoptic operative report for lung cancer surgery
  - Section 1: EMR Autopopulated Information
  - Section 2: Cancer-Specific Information *(required)*
  - Section 3: Additional Procedure Details
- The synoptic operative report summary template
- Knowledge Platform with explanatory notes

American College of Surgeons Standards References

The following ACS standards references are heavily leveraged throughout the synoptic operative report and Knowledge Platform: *AJCC Cancer Staging Manual, Eighth Edition*; *Operative Standards for Cancer Surgery,* Volume 1; and *Standards for Oncology Registry Entry (STORE) 2023*.

Authors

Chi-Fu Jeffrey Yang, MD, FACS*; Jennifer M. Burg, MD*; John A. Howington, MD, FACS*; Hari B. Keshava, MD*; Anthony W. Kim, MD, FACS*; Linda W. Martin, MD, MPH, FACS*; Valerie W. Rusch, MD, FACS*

Reviewers

Matthew A. Facktor, MD, FACS†; Clinton T. Morgan, MD, PhD†; Nirmal Veeramachaneni, MD, FACS†

Contributors

Khalid Amer, MBBS, FRCS (C Th); Frank A. Baciewicz Jr, MD, FACS; Thomas L. Bauer II, MD, FACS; Mark F. Berry, MD, MHS; Matthew G. Blum, MD, FACS; Raphael Bueno, MD, FACS; Lucian R. Chirieac, MD; Traves Crabtree, MD, FACS; Malcolm M. DeCamp, MD, FACS; Todd L. Demmy, MD, FACS; Marc de Perrot, MD, MSc; Jean Deslauriers, MD, FRCSC (C); Frank Detterbeck, MD, FACS, FCCP; Jessica Donington, MD, FACS; Mark K. Ferguson, MD, FACS; Felix G. Fernandez, MD, FACS; Sean C. Grondin, MD, MPH, FRCSC, FACS; Mark Hennon, MD, FACS; Rodney J. Landreneau, MD; Michael Lanuti, MD, FACS; Moishe Liberman, MD, PhD; Jules Lin, MD, FACS; Bryan Meyers, MD, MPH, FACS; Sudish C. Murthy, MD, PhD, FACS, FCCP; Basil Nasir, MBBCh; Varun Puri, MD, MSCI, FACS; Joe B. Putnam Jr, MD, FACS; Rishindra M. Reddy, MD, FACS; Stacey Su, MD, FACS; Betty C. Tong, MD, MHS, FACS; Dennis Wigle, MD, PhD, FACS; Douglas E. Wood, MD, FACS, FRCSEd (ad hom); Kazuhiro Yasufuku, MD, PhD

**Denotes primary author. †Denotes synoptic operative report reviewer.*

Synoptic Operative Report

What This Synoptic Operative Report Covers and Includes
This synoptic operative report (SOR) covers lung cancer surgery documentation.

The SOR includes roughly 15 fields for EMR autopopulated data, 13 fields for cancer-specific data *(required)*, and 15 fields for additional procedure data that assist with billing and regulatory and practice requirements. This synoptic operative report was designed for cases of pulmonary resection for either benign or malignant lesions of the lung. However, narrative text boxes may facilitate expanded use of this synoptic report at the user's discretion.

How This Synoptic Operative Report Is Organized
Required fields are indicated by an asterisk (*).

Section 1: EMR Autopopulated Information

Patient Name*
Patient ID*
Date of Surgery*
Name of Surgeon*
Name of Co-Surgeon
Name of Assistant(s)
Indication for Surgery*
Preoperative Diagnosis*
Postoperative Diagnosis*
Procedure(s) Performed*
Specimens Removed
Type of Anesthesia
Estimated Blood Loss
Drain/Implant
Additional Administrative Details

Section 2: Cancer-Specific Information *(required)*

Indication*
Preoperative Therapy*
Intent of Surgery*
Mediastinal Staging (Mediastinoscopy, EBUS/EUS)*
Location*
Additional Findings*
Pulmonary Resection*
Intraoperative Margin Assessment (By Frozen Section)*
Additional Specimens Sent to Pathology*
Hilar and Peribronchial Lymph Node Assessment*
Mediastinal Lymph Node Assessment*
Additional Components of Resection*
Other Intraoperative Findings*

Section 3: Additional Procedure Details

Approach
Cardiopulmonary Support Used
Bronchoscopy
Analgesia Used
Closure
Soft Tissue Flap Use
Drains
Additional Procedure Details
Intraoperative Complications

Instructions

This report is intended for documentation at the completion of each surgical procedure.

Instructions are provided for each data field.

Explanatory notes provide reference material for each data field.

Narrative boxes are available in all sections of the SOR to allow the addition of provider-specific information as needed.

Completing all applicable data fields in the SOR will generate a SOR summary that is compliant with multiple regulatory requirements.

- **Section 1 Instructions:** You are being asked to review all the data fields in Section 1 as the information is autopopulated from the EMR and should be checked for accuracy. Please make corrections as needed and be sure to complete required fields. Throughout the tool, required fields are marked with an asterisk (*) and represent best practice.
- **Section 2 Instructions:** You are asked to complete all data fields in this section (Cancer-Specific Information) because they are required as best practice.
- **Section 3 Instructions:** You are not required to complete these data fields, but the additional surgical data elements included in this section (Additional Procedure Details) will support diverse coding, regulatory, and practice needs.

Section 1: EMR Autopopulated Information (Note A)

Patient Name*
Patient ID*
Date of Surgery*
Name of Surgeon*
Name of Co-Surgeon
Name of Assistant(s)
Indication for Surgery*
Preoperative Diagnosis*
Postoperative Diagnosis*
Procedure(s) Performed*
Specimens Removed
Type of Anesthesia
Estimated Blood Loss
Drain/Implant
Additional Administrative Details

Section 2: Cancer-Specific Information (Note B)

Preoperative Assessment

*** Indication** (Note C)
Select single best answer.
__ Non-small cell lung cancer
__ Small cell lung cancer
__ Carcinoid tumor
__ Solitary lung nodule (≤3 cm)
__ Multiple lung nodules (≤3 cm)
__ Lung mass (>3 cm)
__ Metastases—Describe whether primary/secondary [*Narrative Box*]
__ Other [*Narrative Box*]

*** Preoperative Therapy** (Note D)
Select all that apply.
__ None
__ Systemic therapy (including chemotherapy, targeted therapy, immunotherapy, endocrine [hormonal] therapy, etc.)
__ Radiation therapy (including chemoradiation)
__ Other/Comments [*Narrative Box*]

*** Intent of Surgery** (Note E)
Was the operation performed for curative intent? Select single best answer.
__ Yes
__ No
  [If "No" is selected, display the following:]
  Select single best answer.
  __ Diagnostic intent [*Narrative Box*]
  __ Staging intent [*Narrative Box*]
  __ Palliative intent [*Narrative Box*]

*** Mediastinal Staging (Mediastinoscopy, EBUS/EUS)** (Note F)
Has invasive mediastinal staging been done separate from resectional procedure? Select single best answer and, if appropriate, add operative description.
__ No
__ Yes—Done previously
  [If "Yes—Done previously" is selected, display the following:]
  __ Bronchoscopically-guided biopsy (EBUS or Navigational/Robotic) [*Narrative Box*]
  __ Mediastinoscopy [*Narrative Box*]
  __ Chamberlain procedure (Anterior Mediastinoscopy) [*Narrative Box*]
  __ EUS [*Narrative Box*]
__ Yes—Done today as part of surgical procedure
  [If "Yes—Done today" is selected, display the following:]
  __ Bronchoscopically-guided biopsy [*Narrative Box*]
    [If "Broncoscopically-guided biopsy" is selected, display the following two fields:]
    Procedure Type
    __ EBUS
    __ Navigational/Robotic

Lymph Nodes Biopsied
__ 2R __ 7 __ 2L
__ 4R __ 4L
__ 10R __ 10L
__ 11R __ 11L
__ 12R __ 12L
__ 13R __ 13L

__ Mediastinoscopy [*Narrative Box*]
[If "Mediastinoscopy" is selected, display the following field:]
Lymph Nodes Biopsied
__ 2R __ 7 __ 2L
__ 4R __ 4L
__ 10R __ 10L

__ Chamberlain procedure (Anterior mediastinoscopy) [*Narrative Box*]
[If "Chamberlain procedure" is selected, display the following field:]
Lymph Nodes Biopsied
__ 5
__ 6
__ EUS [*Narrative Box*]
[If "EUS" is selected, display the following field:]
Lymph Nodes Biopsied
__ 5
__ 6
__ 7
__ 8
__ 9

Intraoperative Findings

*** Location** (Note G)
Select all that apply. If multifocal, each segment should be selected. Indication of specific segments is optional.
__ Right upper lobe
__ Apical segment (S1)
__ Posterior segment (S2)
__ Anterior segment (S3)
__ Right middle lobe
__ Lateral segment (S4)
__ Medial segment (S5)
__ Right lower lobe
__ Superior segment (S6)
__ Medial basilar segment (S7)
__ Anterior basilar segment (S8)
__ Lateral basilar segment (S9)
__ Posterior basilar segment (S10)
__ Left upper lobe
__ Apicoposterior segment (S1+S2)
__ Anterior segment (S3)
__ Superior lingular segment (S4)
__ Inferior lingular segment (S5)

__ Left lower lobe
 __ Superior segment (S6)
 __ Anteromedial segment (S7+S8)
 __ Lateral basilar segment (S9)
 __ Posterior basilar segment (S10)
If more than one, indicate total number of lesions: ______

*** Additional Findings** (Note H)
Select all that apply.
__ None
__ Primary tumor crosses fissure(s)
__ Pleural effusion greater than 10mL
__ Pleural metastases
__ Direct extension into mediastinum
__ Direct extension into chest wall
__ Extensive lysis of adhesions (greater than 60 minutes)
__ Other [*Narrative Box*]

*** Pulmonary Resection** (Note I)
Select all that apply.
__ Wedge resection
 [If "Wedge resection" is selected, display the following three fields:]
 Location
 Select all that apply.
 __ RUL—Provide number of wedge resections [*Narrative Box*]
 __ RML—Provide number of wedge resections [*Narrative Box*]
 __ RLL—Provide number of wedge resections [*Narrative Box*]
 __ LUL—Provide number of wedge resections [*Narrative Box*]
 __ LLL—Provide number of wedge resections [*Narrative Box*]

 Frozen Section
 Select all that apply.
 __ Yes
  __ Cancer
  __ No cancer
 __ No

 Followed by Anatomic Resection
 __ No
 __ Yes [*Narrative Box*]

 Procedure Details
 Describe procedure details.
 [*Narrative Box*]
__ Segmentectomy
 [If "Segmentectomy" is selected, display the following two fields:]
 Segment(s) Resected
 Select all that apply.
 RUL
 __ Apical segment (S1)
 __ Posterior segment (S2)
 __ Anterior segment (S3)

RML
__ Lateral segment (S4)
__ Medial segment (S5)
RLL
__ Superior segment (S6)
__ Medial basilar segment (S7)
__ Anterior basilar segment (S8)
__ Lateral basilar segment (S9)
__ Posterior basilar segment (S10)
LUL
__ Apicoposterior segment (S1+S2)
__ Anterior segment (S3)
__ Superior lingular segment (S4)
__ Inferior lingular segment (S5)
LLL
__ Superior segment (S6)
__ Anteromedial segment (S7+S8)
__ Lateral basilar segment (S9)
__ Posterior basilar segment (S10)

Procedure Details
Describe procedure details.
[*Narrative Box*]

__ Lobectomy
[If "Lobectomy" is selected, display the following two fields:]
Lobe Resected
Select single best answer.
__ RUL
__ RML
__ RLL
__ LUL
__ LLL

Procedure Details
Describe procedure details.
[*Narrative Box*]

__ Sleeve lobectomy
[If "Sleeve lobectomy" is selected, display the following two fields:]
Lobe Resected
Select single best answer.
__ RUL
__ RML
__ RLL
__ LUL
__ LLL

Procedure Details
Describe procedure details.
[*Narrative Box*]

__ Bilobectomy

[If "Bilobectomy" is selected, display the following two fields:]

Lobes Resected

Select all that apply.

__ RUL

__ RML

__ RLL

Procedure Details

Describe procedure details.

[*Narrative Box*]

__ Sleeve bilobectomy

[If "Sleeve bilobectomy" is selected, display the following two fields:]

Lobes Resected

Select all that apply.

__ RUL

__ RML

__ RLL

Procedure Details

Describe procedure details.

[*Narrative Box*]

__ Pneumonectomy

[If "Pneumonectomy" is selected, display the following three fields:]

Lung Resected

Select single best answer.

__ Right

__ Left

Intrapericardial

Select single best answer.

__ Yes

__ No

Procedure Details

Describe procedure details.

[*Narrative Box*]

__ Carinal pneumonectomy

[If "Carinal pneumonectomy" is selected, display the following two fields:]

Lung Resected

Select single best answer.

__ Right

__ Left

Procedure Details

Describe procedure details.

[*Narrative Box*]

*** Intraoperative Margin Assessment (By Frozen Section)** (Note J)
Select all that apply.
__ Bronchial
[If "Bronchial" is selected, display the following:]
__ Positive
__ Negative
__ Vascular
[If "Vascular" is selected, display the following:]
__ Positive
__ Negative
__ Other [*Narrative Box*]
[If "Other" is selected, display the following:]
__ Positive
__ Negative

*** Additional Specimens Sent to Pathology** (Note K)
Select single best answer.
__ None
__ Yes—List all specimens sent to pathology [*Narrative Box*]

*** Hilar and Peribronchial Lymph Node Assessment** (Note L)
Select all that apply.
__ Dissection
__ Sampling
[If either "Dissection" or "Sampling" is selected, display the following:]
Station(s) Assessed

__ 10R	__ 10L
__ 11R	__ 11L
__ 12R	__ 12L
__ 13R	__ 13L
__ 14R	__ 14L

__ None

*** Mediastinal Lymph Node Assessment** (Note M)
Select all that apply.
__ Dissection
__ Sampling
[If either "Dissection" or "Sampling" is selected, display the following:]
Station(s) Assessed

__ 2R	__ 3A	__ 2L
__ 4R	__ 3P	__ 4L
__ 8R	__ 5	__ 8L
__ 9R	__ 6	__ 9L
	__ 7	

__ None

*** Additional Components of Resection** (Note N)
Select single best answer, then select all that apply.
__ No
__ Yes

[If "Yes" is selected, display the following:]
__ Chest wall
[If "Chest wall" is selected, display the following two fields:]
Ribs Resected: __–__

Reconstruction
__ None
__ PTFE
__ Polypropylene mesh
__ Polypropylene mesh and methylmethacrylate
__ Absorbable mesh [*Narrative Box*]
__ Other—Describe implanted material [*Narrative Box*]
__ Diaphragm
[If "Diaphragm" is selected, display the following field:]
Primary Repair
__ Yes
__ No
[If "No" is selected, display the following field:]
Reconstruction
__ Absorbable mesh
__ PTFE
__ Other [*Narrative Box*]
__ Pericardium
[If "Pericardium" is selected, display the following field:]
Primary Repair
__ Yes
__ No
[If "No" is selected, display the following field:]
Reconstruction
__ Absorbable mesh
__ PTFE
__ Other [*Narrative Box*]

*** Other Intraoperative Findings** (Note O)
Select single best answer.
__ None
__ Yes—Describe [*Narrative Box*]

Section 3: Additional Procedure Details (Note P)

Approach (Note Q)
Select single best answer.
__ VATS
__ Robotic
__ Non-robotic
__ Other [*Narrative Box*]
__ Open
__ Thoracotomy
__ Sternotomy
__ VATS with planned thoracotomy [*Narrative Box*]
__ VATS converted to unplanned thoracotomy [*Narrative Box*]
[If "VATS converted to unplanned thoracotomy" is selected, display the following:]

Conversion Reason
__ Vascular (bleeding)
__ Anatomic (e.g., adhesions or aberrant hilar anatomy)
__ Lymph nodes
__ Extent of primary tumor
__ Other [*Narrative Box*]

[If "Open", "VATS with planned thoracotomy", or "VATS converted to unplanned thoracotomy" is selected above, display the following:]
Incision
__ Posterolateral
__ Anterolateral
__ Axillary
__ Hemiclamshell
__ Sternotomy
__ Other [*Narrative Box*]

Cardiopulmonary Support Used (Note R)
Select single best answer.
__ None
__ ECMO [*Narrative Box*]
__ CPB [*Narrative Box*]

Bronchoscopy (Note S)
Select single best answer.
__ Yes—Describe findings [*Narrative Box*]
[If "Yes" is selected, display the following:]
Endobronchial Lesions
__ No
__ Yes [*Narrative Box*]
__ No

Analgesia Used (Note T)
Select all that apply.
__ Intercostal nerve block
__ Paravertebral nerve block
__ Erector spinae plane block
__ Spinal duramorph
__ Epidural
__ Agents used
__ Liposomal Bupivicaine
__ Bupivicaine
__ Lidocaine
__ Ropivicaine

Closure (Note U)
Select single best answer.
__ Normal open [*Narrative Box*]
__ Pericostal sutures [*Narrative Box*]
__ Chest wall muscle sutures [*Narrative Box*]
__ Subcutaneous sutures [*Narrative Box*]
__ Skin closure [*Narrative Box*]

__ Normal VATS [*Narrative Box*]
  __ Chest wall muscle sutures [*Narrative Box*]
  __ Subcutaneous sutures [*Narrative Box*]
  __ Skin closure [*Narrative Box*]
__ Other [*Narrative Box*]

Soft Tissue Flap Use (Note V)
Select single best answer.
__ No
__ Yes
  __ Intercostal muscle
  __ Pericardial fat pad
  __ Thymus
  __ Latissimus
  __ Serratus
  __ Other [*Narrative Box*]

Drains (Note W)
Select all that apply. List size, type, and location.
__ Fr24—Describe location [*Narrative Box*]
__ Fr28—Describe location [*Narrative Box*]
__ Fr32—Describe location [*Narrative Box*]
__ Fr36—Describe location [*Narrative Box*]
__ Other—Describe [*Narrative Box*]

Additional Procedure Details (Note X)
Select single best answer.
__ Yes [*Narrative Box*]
__ No

Intraoperative Complications (Note Y)
Select single best answer.
__ None
__ Yes
  [If "Yes" is selected, display the following:]
  __ Vascular injury
  __ Nerve injury
  __ Bronchial injury
  __ Other [*Narrative Box*]

Synoptic Operative Report Summary Template (Mockup)

Lung Cancer

Patient Name: *[Autopopulate from EMR]*
Patient ID: *[Autopopulate from EMR]*
Date of Surgery: *[Autopopulate from EMR]*
Name of Surgeon: *[Autopopulate from EMR]*
Name of Co-Surgeon: *[Autopopulate from EMR]*
Name of Assistant(s): *[Autopopulate from EMR – Nurses notes]*
Indication for Surgery: *[Autopopulate from EMR; or override with EMR pick list]*
Preoperative Diagnosis: *[Autopopulate from EMR; or override with SOR selections]*
Postoperative Diagnosis: *[Autopopulate from EMR; or override with SOR selections]*
Procedure(s) Performed: *[Autopopulate from EMR; or override with SOR selections]*
Specimens Removed: *[Autopopulate from EMR – Nurses notes with override capability]*
Type of Anesthesia: *[Autopopulate from EMR – Anesthesia with override capability]*
Estimated Blood Loss: *[Autopopulate from EMR – Anesthesia with override capability]*
Drain/Implant *[Autopopulate from EMR – Nurses notes with override capability]*
Additional Administrative Details: *[Autopopulate from EMR; or Narrative text]*

Cancer-Specific Information
Preoperative Assessment
[Fill from SOR: Indication]
[Fill from SOR: Preoperative Therapy]
[Fill from SOR: Intent of Surgery]
[Fill from SOR: Mediastinal Staging (Mediastinoscopy, EBUS/EUS)]
Intraoperative Findings
[Fill from SOR: Location]
[Fill from SOR: Additional Findings]
[Fill from SOR: Pulmonary Resection]
[Fill from SOR: Intraoperative Margin Assessment (By Frozen Section)]
[Fill from SOR: Additional Specimens Sent to Pathology]
[Fill from SOR: Hilar and Peribronchial Lymph Node Assessment]
[Fill from SOR: Mediastinal Lymph Node Assessment]
[Fill from SOR: Additional Components of Resection]
[Fill from SOR: Other Intraoperative Findings]

Additional Procedure Details (Page 2)
[Fill from SOR: Patient Position]
[Fill from SOR: Position Laterality]
[Fill from SOR: Approach]
[Fill from SOR: Cardiopulmonary Support]
[Fill from SOR: Bronchoscopy]
[Fill from SOR: Analgesia Used]
[Fill from SOR: Closure]
[Fill from SOR: Soft Tissue Flap Use]
[Fill from SOR: Drains]
[Fill from SOR: Fluids]
[Fill from SOR: Counts]
[Fill from SOR: Additional Procedure Details]
[Fill from SOR: Intraoperative Complications]
[Fill from SOR: Disposition at End of Operation]
[Fill from SOR: Presence Statement]

Knowledge Platform

Introductory Comments
This protocol is intended to standardize documentation and communication of critical components of lung cancer surgery. The following explanatory notes reference critical elements for cancer surgery as described in the *Operative Standards for Cancer Surgery,* Volume 1.

Instructions

Each Explanatory Note is linked from a corresponding data element in the synoptic report above and contains additional materials and references that can be used to facilitate accurate completion of the report.

Section 1: EMR Autopopulated Information

Note A: EMR Autopopulated Information

Explanatory Comments: The following fields are intended to be pre-populated with site-specific identifiers and information from the EMR.

Patient Name
Patient ID
Date of Surgery
Name of Surgeon
Name of Co-Surgeon
Name of Assistant(s)
Indication for Surgery
Preoperative Diagnosis
Postoperative Diagnosis
Procedure(s) Performed
Specimens Removed
Type of Anesthesia
Estimated Blood Loss
Drain/Implant
Additional Administrative Details

The following table (Table 1) contains the initial FHIR mappings for data fields in section 1, which can be used to create auto-population functionality. Note that FHIR mappings may vary by site and electronic health record (EHR) and will be revised over time.

Table 1. Data Field FHIR Mappings – Lung Cancer (Untested)

SOR Fields	Resource Main Category	Mapping	Version 4.0	Filter Codes Type	Filter Codes	Resource Link	Additional Links
Patient Name	Individual	patient.name	R4			https://hl7.org/fhir/R4/patient-definitions.html#Patient.name	
MRN	Individual	patient.id	R4			https://hl7.org/fhir/R4/resource-definitions.html#Resource.id	
Date of Surgery	Procedure	Procedure.performed[x]	R4	dateTime|Period|string|Age|Range		https://hl7.org/fhir/R4/procedure-definitions.html#Procedure.encounter	See Choice of Data Types for further information about how [x] is used
Name of Surgeon	Scheduling	Appointment.participant.required	R4	SNOMED	1421009	http://hl7.org/fhir/R4/appointment-definitions.html#Appointment.participant.actor	
Name of Co-Surgeon	Scheduling	Appointment.participant.required	R4	SNOMED	1421009	http://hl7.org/fhir/R4/appointment-definitions.html#Appointment.participant.actor	
Name of Assistant(s)	Scheduling	Appointment.participant.required	R4	SNOMED	1421009	http://hl7.org/fhir/R4/appointment-definitions.html#Appointment.participant.actor	
Indication for Surgery	Procedure	Procedure.reasoncode	R4	ICD10	R97.0, R97.1, R97.2, R97.8 R91.8, R91.1	http://hl7.org/fhir/procedure-definitions.html#Procedure.reasonCode	
Preoperative Diagnosis (ICD10)	Condition	Condition.Code	R4	ICD10	C34 – C39	https://hl7.org/fhir/r4/condition-definitions.html#Condition.code	https://hl7.org/fhir/r4/valueset-condition-code.html
Postoperative Diagnosis (ICD10)	Condition	Condition.Code	R4	ICD10	C30 – C39 C46, C45 C78.0 C78.3	https://hl7.org/fhir/r4/condition-definitions.html#Condition.code	
Procedure Performed	Procedure	Procedure.Code	R4	ICD10	G9063 – G9070	https://hl7.org/fhir/R4/valueset-procedure-code.html	
Specimens Removed	Observation Procedure	Observation.specimen DiagnosticReport.specimen	R4	ICD 10 Procedure	31623 31624 31625	https://hl7.org/fhir/R4/procedure-definitions.html#Procedure.reasonReference	https://hl7.org/fhir/R4/observation-definitions.html#Observation.value_x_

Type of Anesthesia	Diagnostic	Observation.code	R4	LOINC	10213-7	https://hl7.org/fhir/R4/valueset-observation-codes.html	
Estimated Blood Loss	Diagnostic	Observation.value	R4	LOINC	59770-8	https://hl7.org/fhir/R4/observation-definitions.html#Observation.value_x_	
Drain/Implant	Procedure	Procedure.focalDevice	R4	ICD 10 Procedure	31643 31626	https://hl7.org/fhir/R4/observation-definitions.html#Observation.value_x_	
Additional Administrative Details	N/A	N/A					
Surgery Location (hidden field)	Procedure	Encounter.location				https://hl7.org/fhir/r4/encounter-definitions.html#Encounter.location	

Section 2: Cancer-Specific Information

Note B: Cancer-Specific Information

Explanatory Comments: This section of the synoptic operative report contains critical oncology data elements supported by evidence and best practice, as well as data fields defined by the STORE manual and submitted to hospital registries for NCDB and state registry reporting. There are data fields in this section related to findings and/or treatments in both the preoperative and intraoperative phases of care. To complete the preoperative data fields assumes that the patient has undergone comprehensive assessment which may include history and physical examination, radiologic assessment, biopsy, and/or staging procedures. For additional details, please refer to the *Operative Standards for Cancer Surgery,* Volume 1, pages 84–86.

Note C: Indication

Explanatory Comments: This protocol pertains to either benign or malignant lesions of the lung. The preoperative cancer type should be selected based on microscopic confirmation of the diagnosis or suspected diagnosis based on preoperative testing. Select the single best option. If the metastases option is selected, describe whether primary or secondary in the narrative box. Indications not listed can be recorded using the "Other" field and associated narrative box.

Note D: Preoperative Therapy

Explanatory Comments: It is important to assess the tumor's response to preoperative chemotherapy and/or radiation therapy. For patients with operable stage II or IIIA lung cancers, preoperative chemotherapy and immunotherapy is generally the recommended approach. Response options are provided for systemic therapy (which includes chemotherapy, targeted therapy, and immunotherapy) as well as radiation therapy (which includes chemoradiation). Other therapies can be recorded using the "Other" field and associated narrative box.

Note E: Intent of Surgery

Explanatory Comments: Intent should be assigned postoperatively by the operating surgeon on the basis of preoperative evaluation and intraoperative management and should be documented as part of the operative report. When the goal is to completely resect the cancer, the operative intent is curative. If the operation was performed for bleeding or symptoms from the cancer, but the goal was not a curative resection, it should be indicated as palliative. Additional response options are provided for diagnostic or staging intent along with narrative boxes.

Note F: Mediastinal Staging (Mediastinoscopy, EBUS/EUS)

Explanatory Comments: In select patients, invasive mediastinal staging may have been performed preoperatively or may be done at the time of index procedure. Indicate whether mediastinal staging was performed preoperatively and use the narrative box to report results of preoperative mediastinal staging if desired.

If mediastinal staging was performed as part of the index operative procedure, select the appropriate procedure and check all nodal stations sampled. Use the narrative box to describe your procedure in detail and/or findings, including frozen pathology results as appropriate.

For additional details on EBUS and EUS, please refer to the *Operative Standards for Cancer Surgery,* Volume 1, pages 97–101.

Note G: Location

Explanatory Comments: Tumor location should be recorded for each focus of disease for which the surgery is being performed. Please indicate the number of lesions. Choose the most detailed location to the best of your ability (i.e., identify the segment, if possible, but lobe is also acceptable if segment is unknown), referencing Figure 1 below. For multifocal disease, please select all locations that apply.

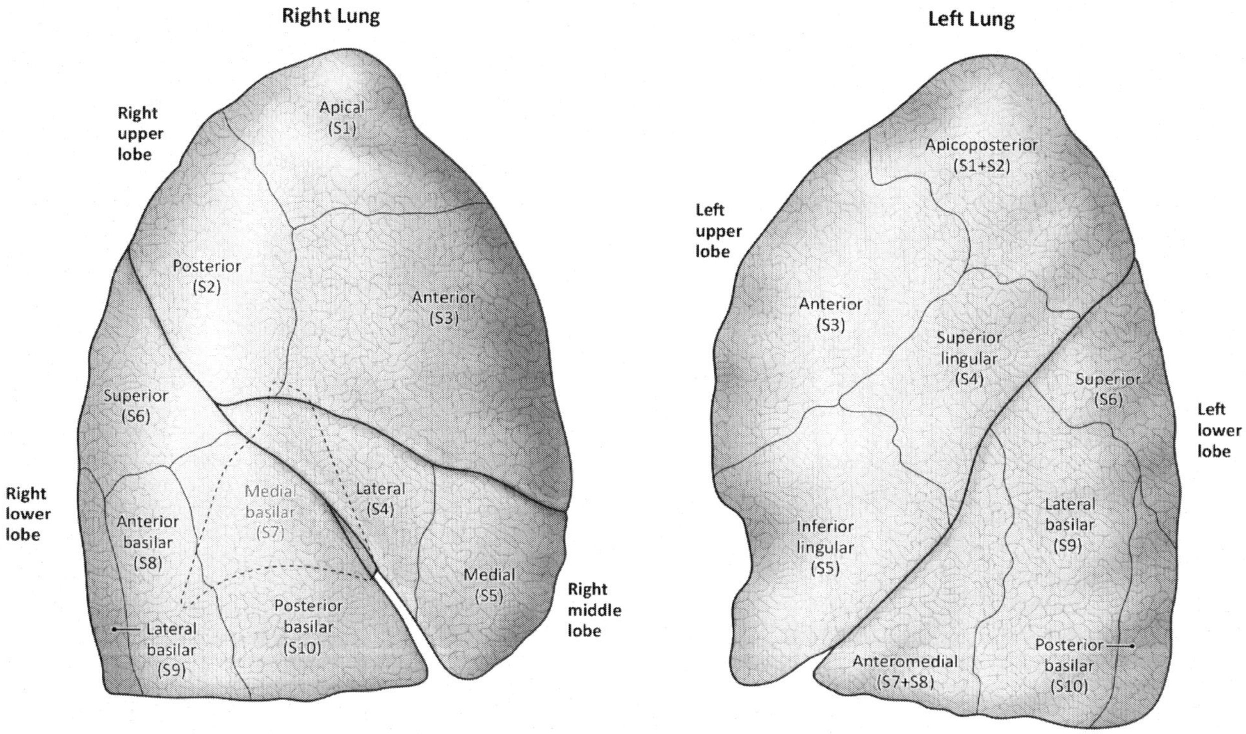

Figure 1. Segments of the lungs.

If relevant, NCDB coding instructions for *Primary Site* [400] are detailed in the STORE 2023 Manual. The primary site is recorded as a "C" preceding the three-digit code number (see Table 2). Laterality must also be coded for lung primaries (see Table 3), following NCDB coding instructions for *Laterality* [410] from the STORE 2023 Manual.

Table 2. Relevant NCDB Codes for Primary Site for Lung

NCDB Code	Definition
C340	Main Bronchus
C341	Upper lobe, lung
C342	Middle lobe, lung (right lung only)
C343	Lower lobe, lung
C348	Overlapping lesion of lung
C349	Lung, NOS

*This table is limited to the scope of this synoptic operative report and does not reflect an exhaustive list of primary site codes for the lung.

Table 3. Relevant NCDB Codes for Laterality

NCDB Code	Definition
0	Organ is not a paired site.
1	Origin of primary is right.
2	Origin of primary is left.
3	Only one side involve, right or left origin not specified.
4	Bilateral involvement at time of diagnosis, lateral origin unknown for a single primary

ACS Standards for Oncology Registry Entry (STORE) 2023. Laterality.
*This table does not include codes 5 or 6 which fall outside the scope of this protocol.

Note H: Additional Findings

Explanatory Comments: Include any additional findings of the case not captured in the above sections including, but not limited to, the findings listed. Please use the "other" selection and the associated narrative box if additional findings critical to the case were present.

Note I: Pulmonary Resection

Explanatory Comments: Select the type of lung resection performed. In the event that more than one type of lung resection was performed in the same case, select all the operations that apply to the case. If a wedge resection was performed, select whether a frozen section was performed for the specimen from the wedge resection.

NCDB coding instructions for *Rx Summ—Surg 2023* [1291] are detailed in the STORE 2023 manual. Site-specific surgery codes for lung can be found in Appendix A and those relevant to this synoptic operative report are summarized below in Table 4.

Table 4. Relevant NCDB Site-Specific Surgery Codes for Lung Adapted from STORE Manual

NCDB Code	Definition
A200	Excision or resection of less than one lobe, NOS
A230	Excision, NOS
A240	Laser excision
A250	Bronchial sleeve resection ONLY
A210	Wedge resection
A220	Segmental resection, including lingulectomy
A300	Resection of lobe or bilobectomy, but less than the whole lung (partial pneumonectomy, NOS)
A320	Bronchial Sleeve resection ONLY Note: A sleeve lobectomy/bilobectomy includes resection of the entire lobe(s) in addition to part of the bronchus. A sleeve lobectomy is distinct from a typical lobectomy or bilobectomy, in which the bronchus is not resected.
A330	Lobectomy WITH mediastinal lymph node dissection **The lymph node dissection should also be coded under Scope of Regional Lymph Node Surgery (NAACCR Item #1292) or Scope of Regional Lymph Node Surgery at This Facility (NAACCR Item #672).**
A450	Lobe or bilobectomy extended, NOS
A460	WITH chest wall
A470	WITH pericardium
A480	WITH diaphragm
A550	Pneumonectomy, NOS
A560	WITH mediastinal lymph node dissection (radical pneumonectomy) **The lymph node dissection should also be coded under Scope of Regional Lymph Node Surgery (NAACCR Item #1292) or Scope of Regional Lymph Node Surgery at This Facility (NAACCR Item #672).**
A650	Extended pneumonectomy NOTE Extended pneumonectomy is the resection of the entire lung in addition to one or more of the following structures: superior vena cava, carina, left atrium, aorta, chest wall, or diaphragm. NOTE: Assign B650 when a pneumonectomy is performed in which the entire lung is removed in addition to part of the carina.
A660	Extended pneumonectomy plus pleura or diaphragm
A700	Extended radical pneumonectomy **The lymph node dissection should also be coded under Scope of Regional Lymph Node Surgery (NAACCR Item #1292) or Scope of Regional Lymph Node Surgery at This Facility (NAACCR Item #672).**
A800	Resection of lung, NOS

ACS Standards for Oncology Registry Entry (STORE) 2023. Appendix A: Site-Specific Surgery Codes, Lung.

Note J: Intraoperative Margin Assessment (By Frozen Section)

Explanatory Comments: Intraoperative evaluation of margin status should be performed and reported using a standard nomenclature following lung resection. Options are provided to report the bronchial, vascular, and other margins (e.g., parenchymal). Each margin that is assessed should be selected and either a positive or negative result should be reported. A "positive" response indicates that invasive cancer was found at the margin.

Note K: Additional Specimens Sent to Pathology

Explanatory Comments: Any additional pathology specimens assessed intraoperatively can be reported using this data item.

Note L: Hilar and Peribronchial Lymph Node Assessment

Explanatory Comments: The hilum and mediastinum should be thoroughly staged at the time of lung resection, even in patients who are undergoing nonanatomic parenchyma-sparing resections such as segmentectomy or wedge resection. On the right side, the sampled or dissected nodes should include the 9R, 8R, 7, 10R, 4R, and 2R nodes. On the left side, the sampled or dissected nodes should include the 9L, 8L, 7, 10L, 6, 5, and 4L nodes and the 2L nodes if accessible. See Figure 2. Preservation of the recurrent laryngeal nerve takes precedence over complete nodal dissection in station 5. For additional details, please refer to the *Operative Standards for Cancer Surgery,* Volume 1, pages 90–96.

Commission on Cancer (CoC) Standard 5.8 requires nodes from at least three distinct mediastinal stations and at least one hilar station to be removed for any curative-intent resection of lung cancer. For full standard details, see *Optimal Resources for Cancer Care (2020 Standards),* page 53.

See also video tutorial on intraoperative node dissection: Operative Standards for Cancer Surgery Video Series | ACS (facs.org)

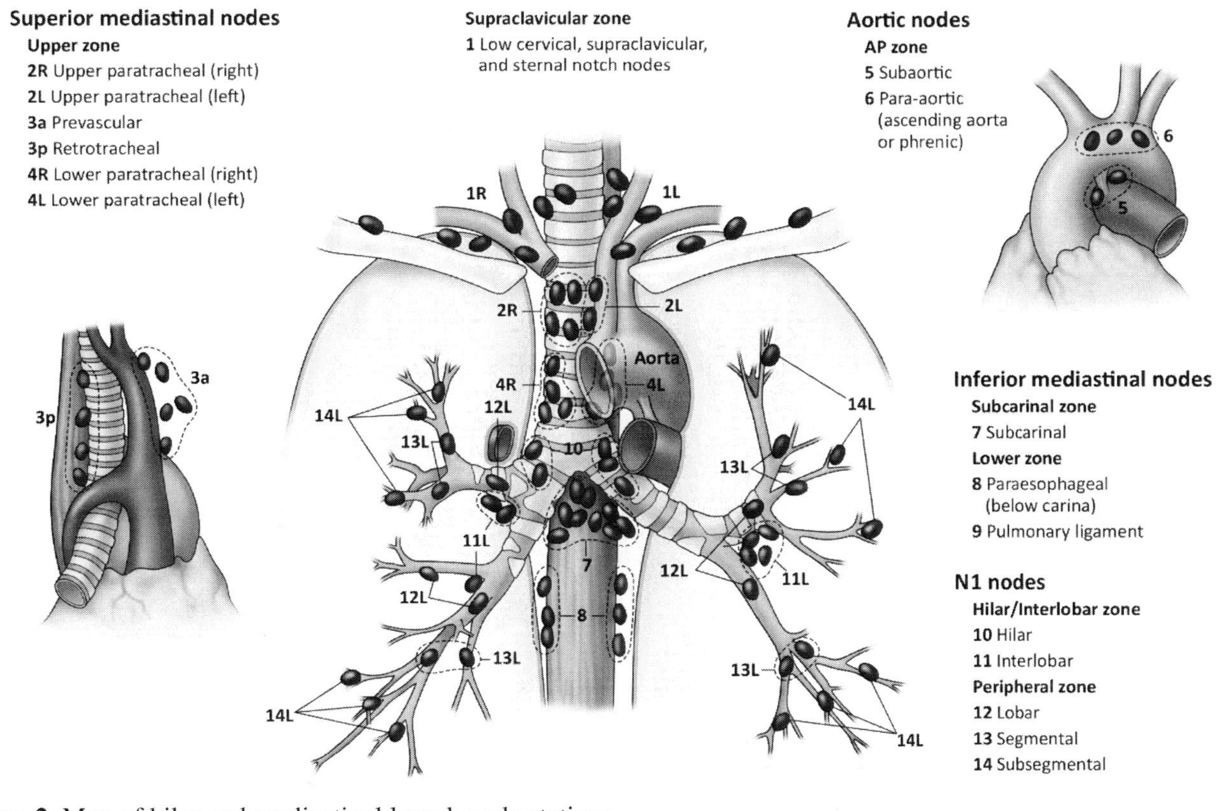

Figure 2. Map of hilar and mediastinal lymph node stations.

NCDB coding instructions for *Scope of Regional Lymph Node Surgery* [1292], used to identify the removal, biopsy, or aspiration of regional lymph node(s) at the time of surgery of the primary site or during a separate surgical event, are detailed in the STORE 2023 manual. NCDB coding instructions for *Scope of Regional Lymph Node Surgery at this Facility* [672] are also detailed on in the STORE 2023 manual.

Note M: Mediastinal Lymph Node Assessment

Explanatory Comments: The hilum and mediastinum should be thoroughly staged at the time of lung resection, even in patients who are undergoing nonanatomic parenchyma-sparing resections such as segmentectomy or wedge resection. On the right side, the sampled or dissected nodes should include the 9R, 8R, 7, 10R, 4R, and 2R nodes. On the left side, the sampled or dissected nodes should include the 9L, 8L, 7, 10L, 6, 5, and 4L nodes and the 2L nodes if accessible. See Figure 2 in Note N. Preservation of the recurrent laryngeal nerve takes precedence over complete nodal dissection in station 5. For additional details, please refer to the *Operative Standards for Cancer Surgery,* Volume 1, pages 90–96.

Commission on Cancer (CoC) Standard 5.8 requires nodes from at least three distinct mediastinal stations and at least one hilar station to be removed for any curative-intent resection of lung cancer. For full standard details, see *Optimal Resources for Cancer Care (2020 Standards),* page 53.

See also video tutorial on intraoperative node dissection: Operative Standards for Cancer Surgery Video Series | ACS (facs.org)

NCDB coding instructions for *Scope of Regional Lymph Node Surgery* [1292], used to identify the removal, biopsy, or aspiration of regional lymph node(s) at the time of surgery of the primary site or during a separate surgical event, are detailed in the STORE 2023 manual. NCDB coding instructions for *Scope of Regional Lymph Node Surgery at this Facility* [672] are also detailed on in the STORE 2023 manual.

Note N: Additional Components of Resection

Explanatory Comments: Describe additional components of the resection for locally invasive tumors, and type of reconstruction if done.

Note O: Other Intraoperative Findings

Explanatory Comments: Describe unexpected findings such as pleural metastases, anatomic variants, blebs or bullae, hilar fibrosis.

Section 3: Additional Procedure Details

Note P: Additional Procedure Details

Explanatory Comments: The following fields have been included for the synoptic operative report to represent a complete record of information so that it will not only fulfill surgeon and institutional documentation needs, but also can fulfill regulatory requirements. The inclusion of open-text narrative fields provides sufficient flexibility for all aspects of surgical care to be recorded and for multiple functions, such as registry submission and generation of billing codes, to be permissible.

Note Q: Approach

Explanatory Comments: The approach to the surgery depends on how the surgery is performed whether open or minimally invasive. If the surgery is performed open, then it should be noted if it is done via a thoracotomy or via a sternotomy. If surgery was performed minimally invasively it should be noted if it is done non-robotic video-assisted surgery (VATS) or robotic VATS. If other minimally invasive techniques are performed, then it should be noted. The criteria for VATS is defined by the protocol published in CALGB 39802. Specifically, VATS shall be defined by no rib spreading, maximum incision size of 8 cm, individual dissection of hilar structures, and a standardized lymph node dissection or sampling. If the operation started as VATS and was converted to a thoracotomy in a planned or unplanned manner, then it should be noted.

Open surgery (whether from the start or if VATS converted to open) shall be noted further by the specific incision used whether posterolateral, anterolateral, axillary, hemiclamshell, sternotomy, or other if one of these incisions was not used.

For VATS cases that have a conversion to open, the major reason for conversion should be noted. Specifically, if the major reason is for bleeding, the "vascular" option should be selected. If there was aberrant anatomy such as an aberrant posterior ascending pulmonary artery branch, then an anatomic reason should be selected. If this aberrant anatomy caused bleeding, anatomic reason should be checked. If it was large, calcific lymph nodes or lymph nodes that made a VATS approach prohibitive, then the "lymph node" option should be selected. If the primary tumor was large or made a VATS approach prohibitive, then "Extent of primary tumor" option should be selected. The "other" option should be selected if the reason for conversion to open is not captured by the other options.

NCDB codes are provided below in Table 5 for the *Approach – Surgery of the Primary Site at this Facility (RxHospSurgApp 2010)* [668] data item from STORE 2023.

Table 5. NCDB Codes for Approach – Surgery of the Primary Site at this Facility from STORE Manual

NCDB Code	Label
0	No surgical procedure of primary site at this facility; Diagnosed at autopsy
1	Robotic assisted
2	Robotic converted to open
3	Minimally invasive (such as endoscopic or laparoscopic)
4	Minimally invasive (endoscopic or laparoscopic) converted to open
5	Open or approach unspecified

ACS Standards for Oncology Registry Entry (STORE) 2023. Approach – Surgery of the Primary Site at this Facility (RxHospSurgApp 2010).
*This table has been amended to remove code 9 (Unknown whether the surgery was performed at this facility) as it would not be an appropriate code in the context of this report.

Note R: Cardiopulmonary Support Used

Explanatory Comments: The vast majority of lung cancer surgery is done without cardiopulmonary support. However, there are instances where cardiopulmonary support is needed (location of tumor, reconstruction, pulmonary function, etc.). If cardiopulmonary support, whether cardiopulmonary bypass or extracorporeal membrane oxygenation (ECMO), it should be noted along with the reason. Explanatory comments are provided to give further explanation for the reason and type of cardiopulmonary support.

Note S: Bronchoscopy

Explanatory Comments: Select whether a bronchoscopy was performed and describe the findings. If an endobronchial lesion was observed, select 'yes,' and describe the findings.

Note T: Analgesia Used

Explanatory Comments: Several different types of analgesia may be used in the immediate preoperative, intraoperative, and postoperative period. Select all that apply.

Note U: Closure

Explanatory Comments: Different types of closure may be used depending on the type of operation performed. Select all methods of closure that apply to the case.

Note V: Soft Tissue Flap

Explanatory Comments: In the event of a more extensive operation for larger tumors, a soft tissue flap may be used during the case. Select all that apply.

Note W: Drains

Explanatory Comments: Post-operative air leak is common after anatomic lung resection. Pleural chest tube/drains can be used to detect or manage air leaks, blood loss, and/or other causes of pleural drainage. Please indicate whether a chest tube was used and enter additional detail about drain type, location, etc. in the narrative box, as needed.

Note X: Additional Procedure Details

Explanatory Comments: Whether to perform additional surgeries should be individualized based on risk and benefits, and those details can be documented here. Similarly, adjacent structures may be removed, or additional procedures may be performed at the surgeon's discretion in the management of the patient's malignancy. Details can be recorded in the narrative box, as needed.

Note Y: Intraoperative Complications

Explanatory Comments: Intraoperative complications are uncommon, but it is important to document them regardless of whether they are related to focal surgical difficulties or systemic events that may relate to patient positioning, delivery of anesthesia, or other aspects of the surgical procedure.

References

1. Amin MB, Edge SB, Greene FL, et al, eds. *AJCC Cancer Staging Manual*. 8th ed. New York, NY: Springer; 2017.
2. Commission on Cancer. *Optimal Resources for Cancer Care (2020 Standards)*. American College of Surgeons. October 22, 2019. Updated February 2021. https://www.facs.org/quality-programs/cancer/coc/2020-standards
3. Commission on Cancer. *Standards for Oncology Registry Entry (STORE)*. Chicago, IL: American College of Surgeons; 2023.
4. Nelson H, Hunt KK, Veeramachaneni N, et al. *Operative Standards for Cancer Surgery*. Vol 1. Chicago, IL: Wolters Kluwer; 2015.

Made in United States
North Haven, CT
05 November 2026

21767755R00015